Success
is the
Quality
of your
Journey

EXPANDED EDITION

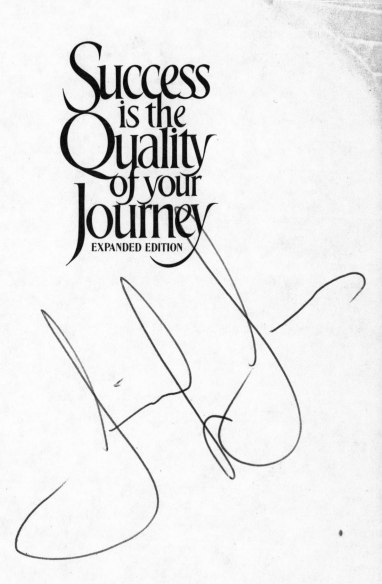

Success is the Quality of your Journey

EXPANDED EDITION

JENNIFER JAMES, Ph.D.

 Newmarket Press • New York

Also by Jennifer James
Visions From the Heart
Windows
You Know I Wouldn't Say This If I Didn't Love You

Copyright © 1983 Jennifer James, Inc.
Revised and expanded edition © 1986 Jennifer James

This book published simultaneously in the United States and in Canada.

7 8 9 0

Library of Congress Cataloging-in-Publication Data
James, Jennifer, 1943–
      Success is the quality of your journey.
      1. Conduct of life. 2. Success. I. Title.
BJ1581.2.J35   1986 158'.1   85-73148
ISBN 0-937858-66-8

Author Speaking Engagements
For information regarding speaking engagements by Jennifer James, contact the author at P.O. Box 337, Seahurst, Washington 98062.

Quantity Purchases
Companies, professional groups, clubs, and other organizations may qualify for special terms when ordering quantities of this title. For information, contact the Special Sales Department, Newmarket Press, 18 East 48th Street, New York, New York 10017. Phone (212) 832-3575.

Manufactured in the United States of America

This book is for you.
Thank you for what you have given to me, to others, and to yourself.

We shall not cease from exploration
And the end of all our exploring
Will be to arrive where we started
And know the place for the first time.

—T.S. ELIOT
"Little Gidding"

Preface
To the Expanded Edition

As I write this the winter solstice has just passed. The days are beginning to lengthen. I am looking toward a new year, the beginning that is part of every ending. It is a fragile time—a twilight—full of both promise and challenge.

I've been caught in all the changes within our culture during the last twenty years. I am stunned by the options available to me yet find it difficult to let go of past expectations. The speed of change in perceptions and values is amazing.

The answers to the age-old questions of "meaning" are now different. We are reminded that we are more than the sum of what we produce; warned that a clean, well-stocked house and a good bank account are no guarantee of joy. We are told that being is more important than having; that reality depends on our perceptions and attitudes as much as on any concrete event or object.

These ideas are powerful, a call to live your life's journey in a different way. You are responsible for yourself and how you feel; for the success and failure of your relationships, and for the condition of the world. You are what you have chosen to be. The future is yours to form. The call for all of us is clear—to be our best selves, to define our existence thoughtfully and to live each moment.

When I started putting the expanded edition of this book together, I had just returned from a journey to Nepal. I felt then a tugging within me that has not gone away, but has only increased. An inner journey is summoning me; I am being tugged and pulled toward light. I have resisted. I have asked for help. I have tried diversions—love, chocolates, and acquisition. I looked for a teacher, a guide, and the answer came loud and clear, like a small explosion in my consciousness. The teacher is within! There will be no hammock this year; there is pulling, not swaying, in my future.

The journey is one toward light, toward grace. Grace emanates outward from the spirit at the center of each person's being. It renders us transparent. We can literally breathe it in when those vulnerable moments come.

From a very young age, I've known it was there in all of us. I looked for it in books, in my church, in my family, and in school. I sought out people who seemed wise or brilliant. Always searching for answers, I turned to Tarot cards, oracles, even the backs of cereal boxes. Bits of information would trigger flashes within me and carry me to the next step. I felt like Alice in Wonderland, getting smaller and larger depending on which cookie I ate.

I became a teacher myself, perhaps to stay close to the world of the scholar, the answers. At the University of Washington Medical School, where I taught for many years, my subject was Culture and Illness—how society and our beliefs make us sick. I discounted my ability as a scholar because much of what I knew was intuitive, not scientific; soft, not hard.

It became clear that academic life was, for me, a way to avoid a real connection with self. As I wrote in "Pop" and "Other Paths," I had to leave the prison of my conditioning and follow my heart. When I began a daily radio broadcast in 1980 and, later, a newspaper column, it was obvious that I was not alone in my quest. The energy was enormous, the love incredible as I gently tested the water, shared my perceptions and listened to "the call."

The essays presented here were originally written for my column in the *Seattle Times* and for my commentaries on KIRO (CBS) television. I started writing them as nudges to myself, quick perceptions and possibilities that helped me to keep things clear. I used to try to draw them as pictures, because that was how they appeared in my mind, but my artistic talents were too limited.

People asked for copies to send to friends. Eventually, I collected a number of the essays and published the first edition of *Success is the Quality of Your Journey* in 1982. We made many mistakes, but sold 10,000 copies almost overnight. Each time we reprinted, changes were made. We learned the elements of publishing the hard way. Three subsequent editions of *Success* were printed and sold out. At that point I was lucky enough to meet the philosopher-president of Newmarket Press, Esther Margolis, who decided to take a chance on a Northwest writer with visions of other ways to be.

There are many paths to the center, but the signposts are all the same—passion, peace, love, and a reverence for life. When you hear or feel "the call," you will follow your path into a new day and, soon, a new century. Remember, when you can, that the definition of success has changed. It is not only survival, the having—it is the quality of every moment of your life, the *being*. Success is not a destination, a place you can ever get to; it is the quality of the journey.

This book is for you on your journey. It is my joy to walk with you.

JENNIFER JAMES, PH.D.
Seattle, Washington
January 1986

*Self-knowledge
is for the purpose
of contributing.*

—ALENE MORIS

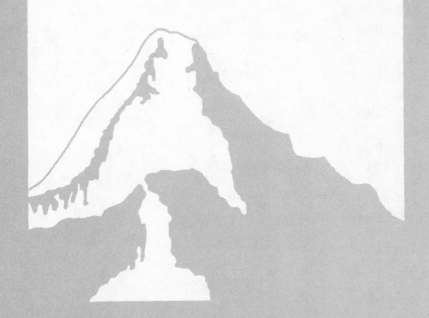

NEW YEAR'S RESOLUTIONS

People are unreasonable, illogical, and self-centered. Love them anyway.

If you do good, people may accuse you of selfish motives. Do good anyway.

If you are successful, you may win false friends and true enemies. Succeed anyway.

The good you do today may be forgotten tomorrow. Do good anyway.

Honesty and transparency make you vulnerable. Be honest and transparent anyway.

What you spend years building may be destroyed overnight. Build anyway.

People who really want help may attack you if you help them. Help them anyway.

Give the world the best you have and you may get hurt. Give the world your best anyway.

The world is full of conflict. Choose peace of mind anyway.

—ANONYMOUS

THE CHILD WITHIN

There is within each of us a child. A child who, to one degree or another, did not receive the parenting he or she wanted. There was not enough love or care or support.

We keep looking for someone to be the good parent, someone to count on. We demand that our own parents change and apologize for their mistakes or inadequacies. They often become defensive and refuse; they didn't have a "total" parent, either.

There is only one way to get superb parenting of the child who will always be within you. Only one person truly knows what that child wants. Only one person will, or can, love and nurture that child to the point of peace and joy. Only one person can be the good mother, father, brother, sister. You are your best parent and friend.

Accept, love, and care for the child within you.

YOU ARE ON YOUR OWN

For the journey of spiritual growth requires courage and initiative and independence of thought and action. While the words of the prophets and the assistance of grace are available, the journey must still be traveled alone. No teacher can carry you there. There are no preset formulas. Rituals are only learning aids, they are not the learning. Eating organic food, saying five Hail Marys before breakfast, praying facing east or west, or going to church on Sunday will not take you to your destination. No words can be said, no teaching can be taught that will relieve spiritual travelers from the necessity of picking their own ways, working out with effort and anxiety their own paths through the unique circumstances of their own lives toward the identification of their individual selves with God.

—M. SCOTT PECK
The Road Less Traveled

DIG DEEP

I painfully dug up the entire field so that I could plant my own crop.

—SHELDON KOPP
*If You See Buddha
on the Road, Kill Him*

Working on self-knowledge is not easy. Often, the harder it is, the more important it is. We dig up things we would rather not see. We resist the pain. We have a choice between a lifetime dull ache and a brief acute confrontation.

We settle for the familiar and confuse boredom with depression.

We all have unexpected moments of insight. *"Oh, that's what that was all about."* Few of us seem willing to push deeper.

People who refuse to do their personal homework reap crops sown in the past by their parents' influence and other powerful experiences. Unwilling to dig deep enough to set their own values and perceptions, they are caught forever working over the same small parts of their past.

Do your homework. Self-knowledge is for the purpose of contributing. You can change your perception of the past to bring peace to your present and our future.

PERSONAL SUCCESS

Some people measure success internally. Others measure it by wealth, appearance, and popularity. Some try to find an internal-external balance.

We're used to establishing our personal scores by comparison. You may define yourself as only the sum of what you purchase or produce. But there is always someone wealthier, more attractive, or more popular. The prize is always just out of reach.

Try a balance or an alternative. Put more time into things with no discernible score. Nurture friendships with people outside your competitive sphere. Walk in the woods, read novels, listen to music, meditate, laugh loudly, play with children and animals, secretly pick up litter, give things away.

Alter your goals to include an investment in the internal quality of each day and in each interaction with a living thing.

You'll win in the long run, if you still want to, because you'll be the prize.

HUMAN POTENTIAL

The human potential movement is big business in the Northwest. They sell millions in books, lectures, seminars, and counseling groups. All of a sudden we have permission to look at ourselves.

We used to call it narcissism or selfishness, but now self-esteem has more credibility.

People are beginning to realize that self-knowledge is not an end in itself. It's for the purpose of better relationships, so that we can give to our community. You can give from overflow. It's very hard to give from emptiness.

The human potential movement encourages us to look at ourselves, examine our values, find out what's truly important to us, change destructive patterns. Some people are afraid; they don't want to take the risk. They think that if they look within, they're going to find some kind of monster. Ignorance is not bliss.

People who avoid self-knowledge cause a great deal of pain to themselves as well as to their families and friends. We now have the permission and some of the information to tap the potential within.

Take your own inner journey, just a few minutes each day.

JEALOUSY

Jealousy is simply and clearly the fear that you do not have value and, therefore, that nothing is safe.

Jealousy scans like a beacon searching for evidence to prove the point—that others will be preferred and rewarded more than you.

Jealousy can be a burning pain, as a particular lover chooses another, or a dull lifetime ache of comparison to everything and everyone.

There is only one alternative—self-value. If you cannot love yourself, you will not believe you are loved. You will always think it's a mistake, or luck. Take your eyes off others and turn the scanner within. Find the seeds of your jealousy, clear the old voices and experiences. Put all the energy into building your personal and emotional security.

Then *you* will be the one others envy, and you can remember the pain and reach out to them.

SELF-WORTH

Some people feel they cannot survive without the support, approval, or love of another person. They decide who that person is and then live for him or her. Sometimes we choose a parent, but it also can be a spouse, a friend, or a child.

You choose dependence because it seems safer. When children were not protected by their parents, they seek protection as adults. They want to be treated like children. You are taught to be dependent by parents or spouses who prefer control to equality.

You may feel worthless, so you use others to remind you of your value. You allow them to be the measure of your worth.

See if you are choosing to let someone else live your life. Then think about what you really want to do. What you want is at least as important as what someone else wants for you, and it's much more likely to bring you happiness.

PERFECT CHRISTMAS

Every year people think about how to have the perfect Christmas, and of course there's no such thing.

What's the perfect Christmas? Is it really necessary to build a tree out of 362 cream puffs? Most of us have one or two things that make us feel Christmas is perfect, but we may not even have time to ask ourselves what they are.

For me, it's being reminded to give to family, to friends, to strangers. But it's also decorating. I love to decorate the house for Christmas and I always give myself some extra time so I can do it.

My stepdaughter likes lots of things, but especially being able to hang her stocking on our chimney. For my husband and his brother, it's being able to cook together.

My brother likes the music and midnight Mass. My sister-in-law likes having all of us together around a table.

What's the perfect Christmas? It may be snow. If that's true for you, drive up to the mountains with your family or friends and get that feeling. It only takes the one or two things that mean the most to you.

Give yourself those things and then save your time and energy to enjoy the feeling of Christmas. There's no such thing as a perfect Christmas unless it's defined by the one thing that's important to you.

PEACE OF MIND

Each of us seeks peace of mind, but we sometimes fear that it means giving up excitement and ecstasy. Peace sounds like contentment, which sounds like settling, letting the fire go out.

Actually, peace of mind allows you to go more deeply into the world and consequently to experience more excitement and ecstasy. The fire burns brighter, fueled by awareness instead of anxiety.

Peace is not something you can force on anything or anyone— much less upon one's own mind. It is like trying to quiet the ocean by pressing upon the waves. Sanity lies in somehow opening to the chaos, allowing anxiety, moving deeply into the tumult, diving deeply in the waves, where underneath, within, peace simply is.

—GERALD MAY

DISGUISES

Halloween is a time of disguises and fantasies. You may prefer not to dress up, but what would you choose to be if you did?

Most women tend to choose something more glamorous than their daily lives. They dress up like movie stars, Marie Antoinette, or ballet dancers. Men tend to be Zorro, weight lifters, or Julius Caesar.

Very few people choose something that's ugly or even scary. It takes a lot of confidence to dress up as a witch or monster. Kids are better at that than we are.

Sometimes we choose to dress as something that we're afraid of. I once thought of dressing as a guru or an evangelist.

When kids come to our door in their disguises, they often want us to guess who they are. They say, *"Can you tell?"* They want us to see them under the disguise.

Adults are that way, too. We dress up as something special, but we want people to see who's really underneath.

GUILT

Guilt is the sum total of:
All the negative feelings we have ever had about ourselves!
Any form of self-hatred, self-rejection, feelings of worthlessness, sinfulness, inferiority, incompetence, failure, or emptiness.
The feeling that there are things in us that are lacking or missing or incomplete.

—DR. KEN WAPNICK

When we hold onto the negative in ourselves it comes with endless guilt. We hold onto a lifetime of floating visions and regrets about what we should have done or should have become.

Conscience recognizes wrong and tries to atone. But guilt turns into resentment. Conscience brings us closer to each other, guilt drives us apart.

Create a new feeling. Every time guilt settles in your stomach, write "I forgive" on a piece of paper. Send it up the chimney, tear it up and flush it, put in the garbage. Don't eat it.

You are not missing anything. You deserve everything.

RETRIBUTION

Fear of success is a common anxiety in our time.

Never mind the definition of success, that's up to you. Let's talk about the fear. Sometimes it's a fear of good news or even personal pleasure. We also fear competition and envy. We refer to luck instead of our hard work.

Have you ever had a supremely happy moment that suddenly darkened, as if your mind were instantly restoring the dark/light balance?

You're driving home after being told you've earned a great promotion and you start imagining your child has been hurt. You're enjoying a wonderful vacation when you start wondering if your house has burned down.

Many people limit pleasure and success with an internal fear of retribution: Someone or something will get me if I'm too happy.

I think it stems, in part, from our old beliefs in animism. We thought the sun god demanded exchanges, so we gave part of our crops and the occasional blood sacrifice. We kept the balance.

Make it safe to feel happy and successful. Let go of the retribution theory of life. Don't administer pain to yourself to maintain a false balance.

The happier you are the more likely you will want to share it with others.

That is the element of balance.

BURNOUT

You know what burnout is—asking too much of yourself, letting go of harmony, devaluing your worth.

Burnout is not only a question of what you do but how you feel about doing it.

UNDERSTAND YOU'RE DOING IT FOR YOURSELF, NOT FOR OTHERS.
You have decided to do this work because of what it does for you.

INVEST IN THE PROCESS, NOT JUST IN GOALS.
Put quality into the steps of your work instead of waiting for a finished product. Don't require that it be perfect for you to feel satisfied.

LET PEOPLE USE YOU.
That's what service is about. As long as you consent, it doesn't matter. When you don't want to do something, say no.

USE STRATEGIES, NOT MODELS.
If what you're doing isn't working, try something else. Models only help when they work.

STOP CARING WHO GETS THE CREDIT.
It wastes time and energy. Sooner or later credit catches up with you all by itself.

GIVE FROM OVERFLOW, NOT FROM EMPTINESS.
Give yourself the compassion and service you are so willing to give others.

UNDERSTAND WHY YOU'RE DOING WHAT YOU'RE DOING.
You have chosen service as a means to reach a deeper understanding of self and life.

Take a deep breath, thank those who give you the opportunity to care. Take care of yourself so you'll have the energy to take care of the rest of us.

LIFEWORK

When the specter of unemployment frightens us, it's easy to forget that lifework is much more than what you can get paid for.

Lifework is many things. It is what you do to maintain your home. It's very important to have a comfortable home. One that pleases you. Lifework is what we do to stretch our creative side, whether as an artist or craftsperson, or through recreation.

It's our work in the community. It's hard to be happy without giving in some way to the world around us. Lifework is also our spiritual journey.

If you know someone who's having trouble finding that ideal job, gently remind him or her of the great scope of lifework. If you are one of those people, expand those parts of your lifework that you do control. Do what you need to do to make money, and create lifework value in other ways.

STRESS

Everyone needs a certain amount of body tension. It keeps us upright. But how much is too much? Have you checked your body lately? How are you feeling? How about your neck, how stiff is it? Or your shoulders? Can you find your balance? Do you feel centered? Are you irritable? Have you yelled at anyone lately? How about your stomach? Your stomach will always tell you the truth, unless you give it antacids and teach it to lie. We know how to tell that we're tense, but we sometimes ignore it. The question is, why?

We know that exercise gives almost instant relief from tension. We know that if we give up caffeine and sugar, stop smoking, give up being workaholics, we can relieve stress. But we don't choose to.

Some people think that someone else will take the responsibility—their parents, their friends, their spouse, maybe even Mother Nature. But if you don't take care of yourself, no one else will. What is your choice? Why are you choosing not to take care of your stress? Do you think that you don't deserve to feel better?

You do.

RANTS

We all have seasons for ranting. Times when there are fewer distractions, and we turn to politics, economics, relationships, and religion. People all around me are ranting about AIDS, the Pope, wealth, and poverty.

I am ranting too, about passion and grace (we need more), about stress (we need less), about people's tendency to threaten other people with religion, about political nastiness, bombing, and kidnapping, and even about the mess left in my hall.

A good, solid rant is great. Some do it in the shower, others behind the wheel, in bars, or at home with those who understand.

Let go of the referee once in a while, let your thoughts and emotions combine in subjective ecstasy. Then take a deep breath, straighten up, smile, and head out to another thoughtful day posing as a rational being.

Inspired by an essay by Lance Morrow, Time *magazine, August 12, 1985.*

DEATH WISH

In the West, we've known about the individual death wish since long before Freud. It's such a prevalent thing that most of us have to guard against it continuously, practically beating it out of our psyches with a stick. Eighty percent of all deaths may actually be suicides. Persons who lack curiosity about life, who are guilt-ridden and depressed and conditioned by parental example, are all too willing, subconsciously, to cooperate with—and attract—disease, accident and violence. . . .

The key to defeating the personal death wish is to genuinely like yourself.

—TOM ROBBINS
"Judy Garland and the Global Death Wish,
or, How to Stop Worrying and Enjoy Stolichnaya"

SELF-LOVE

We receive mixed messages about taking good care of ourselves. Love thy neighbor as thyself means to love thyself *and* thy neighbor.

Yet, self-love often is confused with selfishness and conceit. We are selfish when we do not love and accept ourselves, and attempt to take from others to fill that emptiness.

Conceit indicates low self-worth and an attempt to conceal it. It is difficult to extend to others what you have not been able to give yourself.

Take good care of yourself so you can care about the rest of us.

LONELINESS AND SOLITUDE

We choose solitude. We think loneliness chooses us. People fight loneliness because they think it is a statement about their self-worth, instead of a choice they have made.

You might be lonely because you've defined only a few unavailable or select individuals as worthy companions: your ex-lover or ex-spouse, your adult children, someone who is dead, or someone of your "class" and accomplishments.

You are lonely because you are a discriminating person. There are lots of people available to be with if you are willing to seek them out. Loneliness doesn't choose you, you choose loneliness in preference to the alternatives. There is nothing wrong with your preference—just recognize it and adapt to the circumstances that result.

Solitude is quite different. It is wonderful because you want to be with the person you're with: yourself. You cherish solitude.

The difference between loneliness and solitude is your perception of who you are alone with and who made the choice.

CHILDREN OF LIGHT

No one can give a definition of the soul. But we know what it feels like. The soul is the sense of something higher than ourselves, something that stirs in us thoughts, hopes, and aspirations which go out to the world of goodness, truth and beauty. The soul is a burning desire to breathe in this world of light and never to lose it—to remain children of light.

—ALBERT SCHWEITZER
Reverence for Life

JOY

Joy, bliss, and passion are becoming themes in my speeches at the moment. I'm not sure why. I think it's a reaction against sophistication. Passion and joy are by definition messy. Thrills and tears, laughter and emotional quakes make us damp and wrinkled. Buttons pop off, noses run, hair tangles, glasses slip, and things get dropped and tripped over. Voices shake and the right words are forgotten.

These things never happen if you're sophisticated. When you are cool and elite nothing chips, things stay in their places. Style and perfection can be limiting.

Watch out. If you ever get it all together—nothing but the finest, no scratches, no loose buttons, everything clean— you may not want to run the risk of joy.

BLISS

Bliss break! Bliss break! If even hearing the word *bliss* makes you suspicious or fills you with disdain, let's call it a stress-reduction seminar.

It's time to stop for a few moments of pure pleasure. Time to make a list of a different sort, just so that you remember what turns you on. List all the things that give you a thrill. This thrill is just for you, so exclude anything that requires someone else.

I'll share with you my most recent list:

music (Merle Haggard)
water (playing in it)
anything that grows
perfumes & other smells
catalogs
hotel rooms (just me)
neon
champagne
papaya
street fairs
my new down vest
bulbs in pots (waiting for them to grow)
cloth napkins
sparkle
sushi
peppermint tea
warm socks
solitude
putting my feet up
caffé latte
dreaming
letting go (just being a blob)
heating pad
ferries (round trip)
paperweights with snow inside

    sitting in front of fires
    little oranges
    Christmas concerts
    school pageants

Just making this list excited me. It's true that I'm easy
to thrill. How easy are you to turn on?

MAGIC MEETINGS

We all have problems, but we rarely use our inner resources to solve them.

I occasionally conduct magic meetings. One kind is just a meeting in a meadow with an imaginary woman who is very wise. She is always available to help me if I sit quietly and wait.

Another is a meeting with interesting people. We sit around a table and the guests each give me advice. I invite those who I think have some experience with the problem, and they're always willing to share their knowledge.

Last time, I invited Georgia O'Keeffe, Jane Austen, Steven Spielberg, Alice Walker, Charles Dickens, and Thomas Jefferson.

Try rising above yourself with a group of friends, and gain a new perspective. Whom would you invite to help?

MUSIC

All music is what awakes from you when you are reminded by the instruments.

It is not the violins and the cornets—it is not the oboe nor the beating drums, nor the score of the baritone singer singing his sweet romanza—nor that of the women's chorus,

It is nearer and farther than they.

—WALT WHITMAN
"A Song for Occupations"

SEPTEMBER FEELING

When Labor Day has come and gone, and the children are back in school, some of us get that "September feeling." We feel the letdown as summer slips away.

In spite of the fact that January is the official beginning of the year, I've always felt that September was. We are all keyed in some emotional way to the school year, which so affected us as children. But now no one sets out a curriculum for us, a course of study where our growth can be measured.

The September blues are really a desire to have the potential to start over with new notebooks and a new class.

Start your own new class; set your own goals for what you want to accomplish this fall. As the children start with their new teachers, become your own new teacher.

VISIONS

I live in a part of the country known for visions. Indians who sought to come of age, to make peace with their environment, and to gather strength went on arduous vision quests.

The early part of the year, the quiet before spring, is the perfect time to get in touch with your visions.

Let yourself be aware of what you truly desire. Try to concentrate on your deepest yearnings, not on the surface clutter. You will feel it when your mind and heart resonates within you. You will know what you want.

Write it down and create a vision of receiving what you have asked for. Share your visions with friends to give them the strength of a public presence. Put your will, intent, and support on the same path.

Make an announcement to the universe that you are willing to follow your dreams.

GROWING UP

I used to lie in my bed at Girl Scout Camp on Lake Coeur d'Alene and figure that I'd know what was going on by the time I was 21.

Certainly, I thought when I was 21, I'd have life understood by 25. That was old; I'd be a fool not to know by then.

At 30 I said, "*So this is it. Well, I think I understand.*"

At 33, I kept singing, painfully, the lines from the song, "*What's it all about, Alfie?*"

I felt settled at 35; this must be it. But I found myself revising all I thought I knew at 39.

At 43, I'm about halfway physically, just starting philosophically and spiritually. At peace personally until next week changes me. Just starting to figure it all out.

I'm sure I know when I'll understand it all. It will be at the last moment, well into my 90's, when I draw the final breaths and say to myself, "*Oh, that was it.*"

PURPOSE

There is a cosmic issue, an "inner cosmos" question, always floating about in our universe: Once I have food and shelter, what's next? Where is the meaning? What is my purpose?

Fred Lehrman of the Granite Bay Institute reminded me that our first purpose is the maintenance of our health.

The second is to provide service to others and to enjoy our world and our lives.

The third, perhaps the one we're still confused about, is to check our form. We are the model of the future.

Your assignment is to 1) pay attention to the voice of your mind and body; 2) master something, choose a form in which to excel; and 3) take action, share yourself in any way that pleases you.

When you get stuck, listen to Pablo Casals playing the Schumann cello concerto. Listen to yourself.

All you need lies within.

THE JOURNEY

Success sometimes seems like a collection of products, or a place that you can get to or buy. When we are small we think we will be happy when we can finally turn over or walk or go to school. Then it's being old enough to date or drive or finish school—that really feels like success.

Some people think success is getting married. That's when they'll really be happy. Or that real happiness comes when a baby finally arrives. Maybe we'll be successful and happy when we get that job or promotion, or when the kids finally leave home and we have some peace. Success might be when the house is finished or when we retire. The "golden years"—that's it. That's when we reach success.

Success is every minute you live. It's the process of living. It's stopping for the moments of beauty, of pleasure; the moments of peace. Success is not a destination that you ever reach. Success is the quality of the journey.

LIGHT

One of the hardest things we have to do in life is to pay off our childhood debts, the guilt and defenses developed within our families. Some of us never do, and remain forever prisoners of childhood, with the expectation that others will be the source of light.

If you were a very sensitive child, you probably felt your dependence on others so early and so acutely that you may have lost your vital, genuine self. You split into two selves. One, the child, appeased the parent to assure security. The other, the unique, individual self, put true feelings aside for a safer time.

For many, the pattern continues with a life of playing roles, toeing the line, and staying neutral. A life often characterized as one of quiet desperation.

It is worth the struggle to fight and, with help, to achieve a re-unification of self and a strong link with your vital center.

You are the only source of light.

SEEKERS

Once upon a time, a guru gave a public lecture. He charged $700 for admission and made a money-back guarantee to grant all wishes. The guru posed a question to the crowd of seekers, "When you get what you want, will you really take it?"

He divided the seekers into groups of four and instructed them to discuss their wishes. One group agreed they all wished to feel peaceful.

During a private audience, the guru heard the group's wish. He smiled broadly. "That is easy," he said. "You each can have peace. Now! There is nothing you need to do first to be peaceful; merely accept peace."

But the first seeker shouted, "How can you expect me to accept peace now? Look at the state of the world! Reagan and the Russians are building more and more missiles. I can't be peaceful until every missile is dismantled." He took his money and left feeling angry.

The second seeker whined, "How can you expect me to accept peace now? My ex-husband treated me badly. I can't be peaceful until he gives me the overdue alimony and an apology." She took her money and left feeling cheated.

The third seeker spoke quickly, "How can you expect me to accept peace now? I am in the third year of law school. I can't be peaceful until I pass the Bar and get a job." She took her money and left feeling rushed.

The last seeker remembered the guru's question, "When you get what you want, will you really take it?" The seeker said, "I accept peace now."

The guru returned the $700. He said, "I cannot give you peace. You have it already."

And the seeker left feeling peaceful.

—Sharon Creedon (Rose of Sharon)
"The $700 Guru"

DETACHMENT

There was a time when we admired detachment, even arrogance. Commercials enticed us with models who were cool and appeared not to care.

Some of us believed that the most attractive person was the one who stood aloof, who didn't need anyone. The one who did not make mistakes, who did not show emotions.

We often confuse fear, isolation, and their disguises with independence. We fear genuine emotion and settle for coolness. There is a safety in the lack of intensity.

Yet we always are hoping that someone will see beneath the disguise and cherish what we really are.

You must be touched by life or you are not there. Allow yourself to feel the intensity of being alive, whether it is joy or pain. Share your vulnerability.

PASSION

I'm worried about passion. I recently bought a book entitled *A Passion for Excellence*. It was a big hardbound book with a bright red cover. It was expensive and the words *passion* and *excellence* were emblazoned on the cover in huge letters.

I took it home sure there would be ecstasy hidden inside. It turns out it was a book about business.

Now I'm sure there are a lot of thrills in business, but if we seek passion there it may be because it's lacking elsewhere in our lives, or because we can't tell the difference between passion and anxiety.

Passion doesn't come from business or books or even a connection with another person. It is a connection to your own life force, the world around you and the spirit that connects us all. You are the source.

Books, work, music, people, sunsets all provide sparks, but only you can light the fire.

*Love
comes in simple ways.*

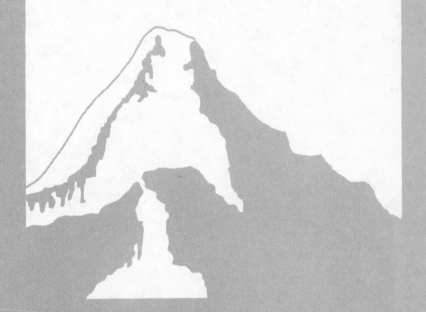

FRIENDSHIP

Friendship is a measure of our ability to love and be loved. Our desire is to feel close and share our life with at least a few others.

Yet some people confuse the number of people they see with friendship.

People build closeness by giving friendship priority, by being honest and showing their feelings. I like to call it being transparent. They communicate warmth, touch, talk about their affection, give each other space, allow change, limit expectations, listen, and offer loyalty and trust.

They avoid trying to control or manipulate their friends. They don't criticize and they don't become dependent.

It takes practice to be a good friend, and we all make mistakes. Friendship, like love, is something you do, something you give that comes back to you.

SECURITY

What do you need to feel safe in the world? It's the same set of skills that children need.

The acceptance of your physical characteristics. Are you careful not to tease children about their physical image? Are you comfortable with yours?

Friendships with people of both sexes. Can you trust both men and women?

Emotional independence. Can you separate yourself from the adults who parented you? Can you survive alone? Do you see yourself as a separate individual? Do you encourage your children to take care of themselves?

Do you have a clear set of personal values? Not values that are an imitation of your parents', but ones you have carefully thought out and chosen to live by?

Are you involved in your community? Some contribution to the larger good is essential to well-being. Children need early involvement in giving and being a part of their community.

Can you stand alone economically? Economic independence is essential to peace of mind.

Parent your children with these thoughts in mind and consider them yourself. A safe personal foundation allows you and them to take risks and to choose a fuller and more creative life.

SHARING

I am frequently asked by women in love, *"How can I build intimacy? He won't talk about personal issues."*

Men have often been the emotional victims of a survival strategy that required toughness, not sensitivity. They were told that their masculinity was more important than their lives. Now that women want men to express a full range of emotions, to show their deep feelings, it's not an easy shift to make.

You can create a safe environment for men to reveal their feelings.

- Be a model yourself—live your life in a sharing, open way. Share your doubts and your understanding.
- Don't blame yourself—it only creates guilt and resentment if you think you're the reason he doesn't talk or share.
- Create a safe environment—accept whatever personal insight is offered, don't correct or criticize.
- Don't make him wrong—this is a time to listen. Choose to be happy, not right.
- Be patient—intimacy takes a lifetime. Sharing of deeply held feelings takes years, even decades. Don't expect it to happen all at once.

We can never truly know another person, but we can make it safe for him to know and share himself.

LOVE

How do we find self-love in the midst of loneliness, depression, feelings of worthlessness? Love for and from others in the face of rejection, absent children, cold marriage, the loss of a love?

The impression is that love is something that happens to you like magic. That love is something others do for you, but that you cannot do for yourself.

Love is not something you wait for. Love doesn't just happen. *Love is something you do.* When you want love, give love.

Moment to moment, you make the choice whether to give love and be loved.

THE ROSE

Some say love, it is a river
  That drowns the tender reed.
Some say love, it is a razor
  That leaves your soul to bleed.
Some say love, it is a hunger,
  An endless, aching need.
I say love, it is a flower,
  And you, its only seed.

It's the heart afraid of breaking
  That never learns to dance.
It's the dream afraid of waking
  That never takes a chance.
It's the one who won't be taken
  Who cannot seem to give.
And the soul afraid of dyin'
  That never learns to live.

When the night has been too lonely
  and the road has been too long;
And you think that love is only
  For the lucky and the strong,
Just remember in the winter,
  Far beneath the bitter snows,
Lies the seed that with the sun's love,
  In the spring becomes the rose.

—Amanda McBroom

49 ❧

PASSION

We all seek passion in our lives, unless we are tired or afraid. But a problem comes when we confuse passion with anxiety.

We mistake passion and desire for fear and tension. The person who doesn't call or doesn't seem to want us becomes more desirable. We feel such relief when the person finally arrives and lets us hold him or her. We confuse relief with desire.

Our romantic culture often describes love in terms of pain. Love, on the contrary, is supposed to feel good. When it doesn't over a period of time, it's probably not love.

Yet in some relationships,, when we feel no anxiety because we are loved, we confuse contentment with boredom. When we feel no tension it seems less interesting.

When you want more passion in your life, the temptation is to find someone else to provide some anxiety. Usually we get more than we bargained for in pain and hurt relationships.

When you want more passion in your life, put more into yourself. If you rely on others, you will always be looking just beyond the relationship you're in. Always hoping there is more.

There is more, always more—but the source is you.

MAKING LOVE STAY

"Why doesn't love stay? Why am I getting divorced? We fell in love and somehow it didn't hold together."

I often think of a relationship as each of us being given an intact heart and a single-hole punch. Now most relationships can take a few holes, and we can patch them up, but too many and it begins to fall apart.

It's easy to put holes in relationships. Do you criticize?— *"You're too fat, you don't earn enough money, I don't like your hair."* Do you find yourself comparing?—*"You aren't as good a cook as my mother, the man I work for at the office is much more intelligent than you are."*

What about expectations?—*"I thought you'd be much more successful than you are."* What about the issue of trust?—*"I have to work late at the office,"* or, *"Gee, honey, I know it's two in the morning but I only stopped off for one beer."* After *we've* punched a certain number of holes in the heart, the relationship begins to disintegrate. You make the choices, you have the punch.

FIRST

Does it matter to you if you're in first place? I understand if you're an athlete or involved in some other competition, but what about in the context of your family? Does it matter there as well?

So many people think they need to be in first place with the one they love. They'd rather lose the love than settle for second or third.

Most people's lifework comes first, so that automatically puts you in second place. Then the children come next, especially if it's a second marriage. I wouldn't want to marry someone who didn't take care of his children. Children need us more than adults do. Then there are brothers and sisters whom the person knew long before he or she met you. You might end up in fourth or fifth place.

You can get so much love in fourth place that it will never occur to you to push for a higher position. It's rarely a problem of his or her not having enough love, it's your ability to be open to love.

Love is not a contest or a competition. Love is all around. There will always be enough for you.

COMPETITION

Competition affects all our lives—whether you think you're winning or losing. Hard times make us tighten up a little in terms of competition. We find ourselves keeping score, wondering who's got more and why.

How do you see the world? As a limited or unlimited pie?

Sometimes you may view the world as a limited pie. If anyone near you expands his piece of the pie, it takes away from yours. It makes you fear other people's success. How do you feel when a friend has a big success? Happy for him or her? Or does your stomach tighten?

Actually, most things are part of an unlimited pie. If other people are successful you can be happy for them. They expand outward from the center of the pie, there is no rim to stop them. They don't take from you.

Competition affects every day of your life. Other people are either friends who offer support, or possible competitors who threaten your score.

SAVINGS

We're surrounded everywhere by advice on how to save money, invest money, and roll over money for better interest rates. Some of you consider yourselves thoughtful, informed money managers, and spend time every day or every week reviewing your portfolios.

Many people buy insurance to cover every possibility. They are protected against fire, flood, accident, the death of others, disability, even "acts of God."

All this care and protection to maintain our financial security. It's important, but there's a flaw here. It is not fate, it is the unpredictability of relationships. Divorce or estrangement costs far more than a bad investment.

Take the same care, time, and energy every day or every week to review your relationship portfolio. Put together a little inner insurance to protect you against the high cost of personal mistakes.

ESTRANGEMENT

One of the painful things in our lives is when we are separated emotionally from someone we love. Close friends may suddenly withdraw without explanation. Relatives can hold grudges that last a lifetime.

What can you do?

First, find a way to eliminate the issue of right or wrong in your own mind. Put the history of the estrangement behind you. Establish as your objective either renewing the closeness, or at least finding peace of mind.

Write a letter to the person that mentions only the future and expresses your love and desire for some contact. When contact occurs, allow no blame or criticism or expectations or demands to pass your lips.

Accept the level of contact that is offered, however minimal, and remember your objective. Be optimistic in what you share and talk about.

Sometimes you will receive no response. You may want to send a similar letter once or twice a year or cards on special days that indicate you care. At some point, remind yourself that you have done the best you can and that it is time to let go, grieve for the loss, and allow yourself peace of mind.

We cannot control other people's choices, but we can offer an open door, look closely at our behavior, and, if need be, accept some losses.

CONTROL

We all want control. We don't just want control over our own lives; we want control over everyone else's as well. It would be so much better if everyone else would just be like us and do what we want them to do.

"If only they would listen."

"If only they wouldn't be so mean or foolish."

We try anger, guilt, withdrawal, criticism—all methods of control to get them to fall into line.

You may be able to get away with controlling children until they leave home or for as long as you pay the bills. It's a contract: I'll give you money if you let me have control.

That might be okay with employees because you are in charge of their paychecks. It's okay with pets because you provide the food and shelter.

It's not okay with anyone else—friends or relatives: You can tell them what you want, you can hope they get the drift, but you have no control over what they do or say.

When you get angry or hurt, check whether you're wishing you had control over someone. Peace of mind requires you to let go of that desire.

Choose acceptance over the illusion of control.

Let go. Choose peace.

RELATIVES

For many people holidays and time with relatives mean wonderful feelings. But for others they do not. The same negative emotions, the same negative patterns, with the same relatives year after year. Sometimes it's the worst part of their holiday. They keep thinking they can make those relatives change.

It is very hard to change these relationships. Your parents had control over you for years and they may not want to give up that control. If you're a parent, you were used to having control over your child, and it's hard to recognize that your child has become an adult.

How can you change these patterns to make your holidays and your relationships with your relatives more positive? You're the only one that can change. You can change your perception of what they've said to you, your perception of particular people, how you respond to them, whether you let yourself get hooked or not.

You're the one who determines whether it's a positive relationship. You can choose peace of mind over conflict.

POWER

It has always been a mystery to me how men can feel themselves honored by the humiliation of their fellow beings.

—GANDHI

We are all tempted by the opportunity to raise our status by lowering someone else's. Do you define your power in relation to others? Do you let racist or sexist remarks pass by you with no comment? Are you sure you can look at someone and define his or her worth on the basis of class and style?

There is an almost irresistible urge to prove our power and worth through comparison. We view power as power over others. The life of Gandhi offers a glimpse of an alternative philosophy. A different use of power.

Thinking about power makes us apprehensive. Power corrupts, power is violence. We forget the difference between power used to manipulate others and power used to empower others.

Power is a neutral force; we control the quality of its use. People who feel their own life force, their internal power, have no need for control over others.

NEGOTIATION

If you want to win, that means someone else has to lose, and he or she doesn't want to. Everyone of us, in everything we do, tries to maximize gain and minimize pain.

Check your negotiation style. Is it win-lose? That's the most familiar style. The only way I can win is if you lose. We carry that to the point where some people even insist the losers admit they've lost. We want them to cry "uncle." It doesn't work very well because they feel so bad that they want to get even.

Another style is lose-lose. If I'm going to lose, I'll make sure that you lose as well. The losers sulk, they withdraw, they plot various ways to sabotage.

A third style—the best choice—is win-win. What can I give to you so I can get what I want? It's an attempt to maximize everyone's gain. To leave everybody feeling that they got something positive. It's the best choice because it works.

ENEMIES

One way to guarantee unhappiness is to believe that you can get everyone to like you.

Yet many people believe that's possible. We are told as children that everyone would like us if we behaved properly. If they don't like us, we feel it's our fault. We put our energy into appealing to people we may not even respect. We reel from the pain of even slight rejections. We try not to make enemies.

There is no life possible without enemies. If you have no enemies, you're not doing anything.

Cherish your enemies: they are a wonderful source of energy and occasional thrills of self-righteousness.

Examine your enemies: make sure they are the right kind of people. Keep worthwhile enemies to about five, and once in a while reevaluate them.

When there are more than five, take one to lunch. Enemies can become friends, often with only slight adjustments. Something drew you together in the first place.

Evaluate your life by the reactions you stimulate in others. Keep them strong, and recognize they are a measure of your commitment, your willingness to take risks, and the quality of your life.

REVENGE

All of us have times when we want revenge. Sometimes it's for small things like being cut off for a parking space, sometimes for big things like losing a job or being rejected through divorce.

Teenagers retaliate with toilet paper on someone's yard; adults retaliate with gossip. We seethe and we plot.

I was once angry, years ago, at a man who had two hundred fancy suits in a custom-made closet. I plotted: I would cut the left arm off of every jacket. He wouldn't notice until he put one on. Of course, I didn't do it.

It's okay to fantasize about throwing paint on people, running over them with a car, mailing them dog poop, or confronting them in public. But it's not okay to do it.

There's a big gap between fantasizing, which feels good, and actually carrying out the revenge. It's the difference between people who are in control of their lives and people who are not.

The best revenge is, of course, a good life. Enjoy yourself, be happy, be successful. It'll drive them crazy—or you can imagine that it does. You'll feel so good you won't care.

HONESTY

The meaning of honesty seems to have changed. An element of grace once existed that helped separate honesty from permission to insult.

Now honesty for some people means saying whatever is on their minds, regardless of whom it may hurt.

These people preface their comments with, *"I hope you won't get mad at me," "Please don't think I'm being critical," "Don't mind if I'm honest," "I'll be candid with you"*—and then they insult you.

Honesty requires more thought than an insult. Most of us think faster than we can talk, so many ideas that flash in our minds never reach our tongues. Thank goodness!

People are able to act their best when they feel valued. Honesty in the form of insults or criticism wears down confidence.

If honesty means being insensitive, check your motivations.

An honest insult may not be as honest as you think.

EMANCIPATION

The push for independence starts around age twelve. Children express this push in different ways. Some will "talk back" or skip school, others run away from home. The child begins to struggle with opposites: the need to have a home, and the need to be independent. How can we help?

Encourage independence as early as possible. Let your children make decisions, do their laundry, handle their finances, wake themselves up, ride the bus, get broken things fixed. Increase their responsibilities as they get older. A twelve-year-old can make doctor or dental appointments.

Listen to yourself as your children grow up. Can you let them make mistakes? Convince them you believe they can take care of themselves?

During their high school years, make a contract about future schooling and support that you're comfortable with. Agree on a time for them to leave home and stick to it.

Emancipation sometimes seems like rejection, but it really is encouragement. Young adults need it now more than ever.

ANGER

Anger is a response that can lead to harm if we don't evaluate what we are upset about. Ask yourself what you are afraid of, as anger is almost always fear in disguise.

If we think something or someone threatens us, we feel fear—fear that we are inadequate, that our lives are out of control, that things won't go our way. Then we fight.

Find out what you're upset about. We rarely are upset for the reason we think.

Figure out what your goal is. What do you want from the power display?

Do something good for yourself at the moment your anger starts. Usually we are most angry when we have not been taking care of ourselves.

CHILDREN

One of the hard things about being a parent is understanding why children misbehave. If we know why, we can discipline more successfully.

Here are some of the possibilities. First of all, *attention*. Whether it's positive or negative, children want to make sure that we notice them. Sibling rivalry is an example. They will fight with each other just to get our attention. Make sure that you're not becoming a cheerleader for opposing teams.

Another possibility is *power*. All children want power, whether they are four or fourteen. But they really don't want to be in control of the house and family. Watch out for power struggles and refuse to participate.

Revenge. Children are very sensitive about justice and fairness. If they think you have been unfair, they may misbehave just to get even. Discipline, but don't retaliate, or you'll be setting a model for revenge.

Feelings of *inadequacy* may be the most important reason for trouble. Children who don't think they are worthwhile may either stop trying or rebel out of fear and anger.

See if you can figure out why your children are misbehaving. It will be much easier to respond in a way that helps, and doesn't hurt.

MARTYRS

Are you giving all your time and energy to someone who doesn't appreciate it?

Do you sometimes think of yourself as a martyr? Does the word "sacrifice" creep into your mind more than just once in a while?

Many people martyr themselves in relationships and no one notices.

My mother did a tremendous amount for all of us and she would admit now that she thought of herself as a martyr. One day she said to my father, *"Godfrey, I work my fingers to the bone for you and what do I get?"* My father answered: *"Well, I guess you get bony fingers."*

Martyrs seem to give a great deal, but no one thanks them, or at least not often enough. The reason is that the martyr's stock-in-trade is guilt—*"I've done so much for you."* Because guilt doesn't feel good, not only do people forget to say "thank you," they usually stay away.

The martyr is furious—*"I've done so much and I've received so little in return."* In fact, martyrs don't give to other people, only to themselves. They just use other people as the foil.

Try caring and loving, and expecting the same in return. Don't opt for suffering in the hope that someday they will recognize how wonderful you are. They won't.

RESCUERS

Some of us are rescuers by nature. We are always willing to try to help someone else, even if it interferes with the enjoyment of our own lives. Sometimes our help may not be particularly useful, however.

If we're willing to accept the weight of other people's problems, maybe they aren't left with any reason to solve them themselves.

It reminds me of a very heavy, big, awkward canvas ball that we used to exercise with in gym classes. Someone would throw it to us—OOFF—and we would hold onto it, but we were supposed to *try* to throw it back.

What happens when we wake children up in the morning long after they are old enough to wake themselves? Or rescue them when they make mistakes, instead of helping them work out their own solutions? Or make explanations for a spouse who is always late or has some other problem? If we are willing to carry the weight and responsibility, then they don't have to.

Throw the ball back. Offer them understanding, offer support, but give them the responsibility. Then they'll be motivated to try to make some choices to deal with their problems.

SLUGS

My view of criticism is that all those nasty remarks are just slugs that someone is trying to unload. The criticizer may have received so many of the slimy things as a child that he or she is still trying to get rid of them. He or she gets up every morning with a bucketful of slugs, looking for victims.

Those who criticize call their remarks teasing, kidding, or constructive. Constructive criticism is just a slug in a tuxedo. The slug carriers don't understand the difference between criticism and encouragement. They mean to hurt and they do.

Resist assuming that all the slugs they hand you are yours. Instead, bury them or give them back. Eliminate their power by laughing. Don't allow slugs; they make you sick. When your stomach hurts after being with someone, you can be sure it's full of slugs.

Start your own slug-burial service to help all of us deplete the world population of nasties such as *"I'm only telling you this because I care about you."* Disintegrate them with laughter. A slug can easily be giggled to death.

Learn to recognize, bury, hand back, or disintegrate slugs before they get to your stomach.

IMITATION

If a child lives with criticism, he learns to condemn.
If a child lives with hostility, he learns to fight.
If a child lives with abuse, he learns to hurt others.
If a child lives with encouragement, he learns to be confident.
If a child lives with fairness, he learns to be just.
If a child lives with tolerance, he learns to be patient.
If a child lives with approval, he learns to like himself.
If a child lives with love, he learns to find love in the world.

—ANONYMOUS

THE RIGHT WAY

Would you rather be right or happy? That's an absurd question, isn't it? But you cannot be both very often. A lot of people argue about who's right. The right way to roll socks. The right way to open a can.

You're in a car. You're the passenger. Your spouse is driving. *"Dear, did you mean to make that left turn?"* *"Yep, always go this way."* *"Well, you know that's not the best route."* *"I think it's the best route. I think it's the right route."* *"Well, dear, we're going to be late."*

Now if you're smart, you'll stop talking right then because there are two right routes, at least. There's the one that your spouse knows that always gets him or her there, and there's the one you want. But even if you stop talking you may sit there and seethe, *"That fool thinks this is the right way."*

By the time you get to the party or the meeting, you two may be snarling at each other. What's the right way? There are probably about twenty-five right routes from here to there. So next time you're in a navigation argument, if you're not driving, keep quiet. The person who's driving gets to choose the right route, and you get to choose to be happy.

HUMOR

If you could choose one characteristic that would get you through life, choose a sense of humor. Any kind of humor—puns, dumb stuff, gallows humor. A sense of the absurdity of life, even at your darkest moments.

I have a friend who recently had to have a mastectomy—it was scary. She's very young, an actress, unmarried, and there was the possibility that the cancer might have spread. She's a wonderful person with a great sense of the absurd.

I was with her when she came out of the anesthesia. She was still groggy, and the first thing she said to me was, *"Now I have Idge."* I said, *"Idge? What do you mean by Idge?"* *"Well,"* she said, *"they took Cleve."* I laughed and I cried at the same time.

Let people find humor where they can and join them. There will always be enough things in life to be serious about.

ILLUSION

When Thanksgiving comes some people are able to celebrate, but other people turn into martyrs. They spend weeks cleaning the house to make it perfect, and they spend eight or ten hours cooking.

Why do we chase the illusion of the perfect holiday? I think in part it's some of the images in the media. Think of the Norman Rockwell print—it's a classic. Rockwell's painting shows a wonderful Thanksgiving dinner. All the relatives are smiling. The beautiful table is laden with food.

I've tried to put those kinds of Thanksgivings together, but they never look like the picture. They don't sound like it either. I finally realized that the painting is an illusion because there's no audio. For just a minute let's plug a speaker into that Thanksgiving print.

"Well, if you'd put the turkey in on time, George wouldn't be drunk." "I don't know why you cooked sweet potatoes, no one ever eats them." "Tell me, does little Freddy still wet the bed?"

This Thanksgiving don't try for the illusion of perfection. Instead, save some of your energy to enjoy the people with whom you're spending Thanksgiving.

PRESENTS

Have you ever been disappointed by the way someone remembered your birthday or anniversary? Have you anticipated a special present for Christmas and then had to conceal your disappointment when you opened the box?

Disappointment that turns to resentment. *"Why don't they care about me? Why aren't they more aware of my needs and preferences? Why won't they love me the way I want to be loved?"*

They love you the only way they know how: their way. Are you able to recognize and accept other people's styles of loving?

You can always try to teach people to love you in your style, but never expect anyone, no matter how close, to read your mind and heart. Tell them what you want. The investment you make in surprise is often a hidden expectation that brings disappointment.

Better yet, buy yourself your heart's desire. Don't turn special days into tests of love. Take care of yourself in the style you prefer—yours. Then, anything else you receive on that day will seem like extra love that you can enjoy without hurtful expectations.

PERFECTION

Our culture has a serious mental health problem: perfectionism. The belief in the illusion of perfectibility.

A perfectionist's inability to accept human frailty and error causes serious emotional problems.

Adult perfectionism has its roots in unrealistic parental demands and conditional love. You will be loved only if you perform.

Parents who are never satisfied with their children's accomplishments raise children who are never satisfied with themselves.

The issue is not high standards, which we all would support. The issue is a pattern destructive to health and relationships.

Perfectionists can change. See if you can identify the critical voice in your head. Try to be less competitive. Stop keeping score.

Try not to pass it along to others, especially your children. You may find that if you allow others more consideration, you may also be able to give some to yourself.

HEROES

We live in a culture with high expectations for the individual. The sky's the limit!

Most of us are told as children that it is possible to achieve any goal. Sometimes we use other people as models to establish and reach goals. We usually want models who we think have reached the pinnacle of perfection. Their image spurs us on.

Whom do you admire? Are they reachable people, or people you've never met? Are you able to keep them in their place as heroes, or do they slowly crumble the more you find out about their lives?

To find or be a hero is hard. The press will examine every pore. The Internal Revenue Service will examine every figure. There is a tug of war both to place the person on the pedestal and to pull him or her off of it.

Instead of heroes, try choosing characteristics or specific accomplishments to admire. Let parts of yourself and other people be exalted.

Accept that there is a balance in most people between assets and liabilities.

Admire real people. Some will live next door, some will live in the media, but their mistakes and human qualities will teach us as much as their accomplishments.

FACES

Our faces not only reveal our own feelings, they also act as a mirror for other people. What others see in our faces, especially if they are children, is what they project at that moment in time.

What mirror do you offer children? What of themselves do they see in your response to them? What mirror do you offer others? We reflect what we feel. We feel what we are. We are what we believe about ourselves.

Sometimes we see love in ourselves and others. Sometimes we see meanness. Sometimes we see carelessness or failure. Sometimes we see acceptance. Check your reflections.

Cultivate transparency so others can see within you and know that what they see is what you both are.

WINTER

One of the benefits of my job is that I get to wish lots of people Merry Christmas. I'm sitting here Christmas Eve and thinking that for me candles are one of the many symbols of this night. They add light at the darkest time of the year. They represent the spirit. The whole idea of Christmas is the birth of Christ.

It symbolizes for each of us, whether Christian or not, the possibility of rebirth, the winter before the spring. We are reminded how we can add more quality to our lives. We are told to be more tolerant, to be more compassionate, to be more generous, to give to our family, our friends, our community, to draw our family close around us.

Now, it's hard to find all these messages under all the presents and the decorations and all the food, but they're there. You still have a lot of time. There are an infinite number of acts of kindness that are possible within your family and friends.

Let the kids make a few more mistakes; be less critical; put your arms around someone from whom you may be a little estranged. Make peace within your family.

There are many possibilities for those acts of kindness. That's what Christmas is all about—acts of kindness that will stay with us all year long.

BUS STOPS

A young man I know has fought hard to keep his sanity amid the pressure from the world and his family for perfection and success.

He always found it difficult to stand at bus stops because he was sure that he looked weird. People would know he wasn't "normal."

The last time we talked I asked him to make a list of all the "successful" people he knew who wouldn't pass the bus-stop test. He came up with fifty-nine names. Here are my favorites from his list—add yours.

Mick Jagger
Rod Stewart
Luciano Pavorotti
Willie Nelson
Dolly Parton
Jack Nicholson
Art Buchwald
Lucille Ball
Mother Theresa
Sigmund Freud
Albert Einstein
Alexander Graham Bell
Rodney Dangerfield
Larry Bird
Helen Keller
Madonna
Gandhi
Moses
Moshe Dayan
Beethoven
Socrates
Pope John Paul II
Andy Warhol

Next time you're at a bus stop, try to keep your judgments where they belong, tucked inside with all the other prejudices you're trying to let go of. Then smile at everyone. One of them may be my friend.

PERCEPTION

We live in a world of events, . . . [and] our lives are affected by these events because of the way we see them. This is also true of people.

People are to us the way we perceive them. Our perceptions are based on qualities that we are not happy with in ourselves—qualities that we use as a means of making a judgment.

As long as you see someone as a problem, you must remain in these circumstances so you can be "right" about him or her.

It is only when you are willing to allow people to be as they see themselves, without your judgment, that you can free yourself from these circumstances.

—REVEREND ERNIE FORKS
Columnist for *The New Times*

*The only thing
that is certain
for man is change.*

—LEO BUSCAGLIA

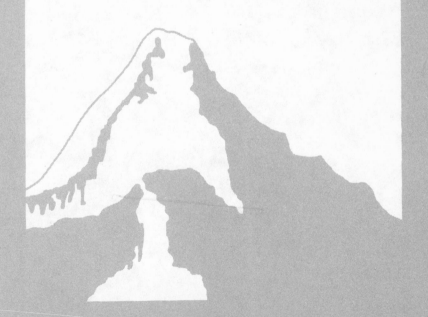

CHANGE

Change is very hard, whether it's an individual desire or a culture-wide need. We prefer the familiar, the known, and we give it value because of that.

We avoid change. We deny what we know in our bones. We block experiences, we ignore intuition, we pass by insight, we avoid transformation. We hold on, afraid to change a pattern even when we are in pain.

When you feel conflict, pain, tension, fear, or confusion, this is a change trying to happen. Don't avoid it or withdraw. Don't turn to busyness or denial. Lean into the feeling, work on the change, take the risk. It will give your life the fullness you seek.

OPTIMISM

As we move into a new year, we have the choice to see it as an optimist or as a pessimist. Do you see weeds or do you see flowers? Is the glass half empty or is it half full? How do you see the world?

Optimists and pessimists think that they base their perceptions on fact, but it's more likely that they are inherited. If you have an optimistic parent, you're more likely to be optimistic. But the filters that color your perception can be changed.

You can look forward to an optimistic New Year. If you're in a traffic jam, remind yourself that you need time to think. If you're sick, you can use the time to decide what's important to you. If you're having economic difficulties, they will force you to reevaluate your priorities. You may end up happier.

Look for the positive hidden in the negative and make a resolution for an optimistic New Year.

WEATHER

Winter is a time of gray, velvet weather drifting toward us. It arrives on "little cat feet" and curls itself around us like the fog in Sandburg's poem.

I'm English and Welsh by birth, so the mist seems somehow right to me, peaceful and snug. The English make gray skies a treat because you can stay inside by the fire drinking tea.

The weather is a friend if you make it one. I look forward to the gray, quiet time for solitude, contemplation, reading, long conversations with friends. Colors are softer, sounds have more depth, the pace is gentler.

Instead of resentment at the lack of sun, snuggle into the gray velvet quilt and ring the butler for a cup of tea. Ask him to stoke the fire and bring you the seed catalogs and travel brochures.

VACATION

We often pile a lot of expectations into just two weeks. If even one day goes wrong, we're disappointed. One of the problems is that we always assume that our friends and family are going to behave differently because they're on vacation. Chances are they'll behave pretty much the way they do at home, and you need to plan for it.

First of all, don't over-schedule. Too many activities mean that you'll be exhausted and somebody will be resentful. At the same time, don't have too few activities. If there's too much free time, someone will get bored and pick a fight. Make sure that you have time alone. Whether you're with friends or spouse or children, a vacation means that you should get some time alone.

If you're going to be roughing it, camping or staying in a cabin, work out the division of labor before you leave home. Otherwise you may end up doing all the work and you'll resent it, and you'll let everyone know that you resent it as well.

Check your past experience. What's worked in the past? Which vacations were good? What were some of the mistakes? Learn from them and then you don't have to repeat those mistakes. Change your expectations. Don't try to do everything for everybody. A vacation means that you get a chance to relax. That's what it's all about.

SMALL FRUSTRATIONS

One of the things that adds tension to our lives is small frustrations. Losing car keys can give you a panic attack. Not being able to find a comb when you get out of the shower, losing scissors and nail clippers, can make you fight with your roommate. The problem is that we think that these things are not supposed to happen to us. And that's what makes us tense.

We think we can avoid these frustrations by making ourselves and others be more careful. I like to take the opposite tack—to assume that these things are a part of life and that they will happen no matter what. Each one of us has a certain quota. You're going to go through 150 combs in a lifetime, no matter whom you live with. So wait for a sale and buy two dozen; then you only have to face the frustration once a year. It's the same with scissors, nail clippers, car keys, wallets, dead batteries, and flat tires. Let's say the quota is eleven lost wallets in a lifetime.

You can do some prevention, but if you assign yourself a quota, instead of tension and frustration, you can say, *"Oh oh, here's number eleven,"* and use your sense of humor.

THE PAST

Everywhere we turn someone or something is telling us to examine our past, to get to know ourselves, to come to terms with our past. Sometimes it's hard to see the relevance. What's done is done. We can't change anything.

Actually we do change the way we view things that have happened in the past. Can you remember how you used to tell your life story when you were about twenty? You'd go out on a date and your companion would ask about you. It might take hours or days. And then when you get to be forty and someone asks you to tell your life story, it only takes a few minutes. The important elements have changed.

Sometimes we change our perception of a specific event. For example, if you got divorced or fired, you might have originally described it as the worst thing that ever happened to you. And now you might be describing it as the best thing that ever happened to you.

You are always free to choose a different past or a different future.

—RICHARD BACH
Illusions

GRADUATION

The important messages are very simple, but most of us don't even start figuring them out until we're past forty. Pain and time are great teachers. We want to share information with our children, because we are hoping they will avoid some of our mistakes. If they take better care of themselves, then they will end up taking better care of us. Here are a few clichés for the future:

First of all, *there is more to life than increasing its speed.* Sometimes we move so fast after quantity, that we forget about quality. Another one, *if at first you don't succeed, you're running about average.* Sometimes we set up so many expectations for ourselves that we declare ourselves failures before even starting.

Your growth and wisdom can be directly gauged to the drop in your ill temper. There are a lot of grouches out there who are impatient and critical and pessimistic. Wisdom is much more likely to be connected with optimism and an even temper. *Like yourself now. Be ten years ahead of your friends.* I wish someone had told me that. *There are very few things that are truly important.*

Remember, you decide what's truly important by your own values. You make the choices, no one else does. You're always going to be learning. You're always going to be continuing on your journey.

Graduation is only the recognition that you've taken a big step.

QUALITY

We're often being told to take care of ourselves by people we don't even know. I remind you to reduce stress. I tell you to choose peace of mind, but I don't always follow my own advice.

One of the things that helps me is a rule to always try to choose quality over quantity. If you're not feeling satisfied, if you don't feel centered, if you think you're moving too fast, take a minute, take a piece of paper and make two columns. One you can call quality and the other, quantity.

Re-evaluate your week. How did you spend your time? What kind of choices did you make? In terms of relationships, did you choose quantity or quality? What about food? Did you choose quantity? Purchases that you made, decisions that you made—what was your choice? In how many things did you choose quantity and how many quality?

Once you can see the balance in your life you can make small shifts. You'll feel the difference.

PERFECTIONISM

Reaching for the stars, perfectionists may end up clutching air. They suffer from mood disorders, troubled relationships, and stress. They may even achieve less than others.

—DAVID BURNS

The healthy pursuit of excellence, the genuine pleasure of meeting high standards, is often confused with perfectionism.

Perfectionism is based on a painful illusion, the illusion of personal perfectibility, people measured entirely by production or accomplishment.

Perfectionists lose sight of the quality of life in their search for quantity. Order ends up taking precedence over relationships. Their expectations are more important than acceptance and love. They can see only perfect and imperfect, so they are unable to enjoy any activity or person that would leave them in between.

Perfect performance becomes confused with perfect love. They are never satisfied. They never really feel safe or loved.

Sometimes perfectionists give up and become total failures. Some feel inadequate, but try to conceal it by demanding perfection from others. Some procrastinate, afraid to make mistakes. Some choose suicide to avoid the inevitable failure of maintaining the illusion.

Recognize perfection as an illusion, not a desirable way to live. Don't confuse it with excellence. Enjoy your successes, laugh at your failures and learn from them. Relax, become less competitive and critical. Enjoy life instead of controlling it.

TEXTURE

Each of us makes the choice about how we feel, though it often seems to be controlled by other people or events. We can alter our perception. We can restore our balance. We can choose peace of mind. We can choose the texture of a day.

Each day seems to have a life of its own, but we are that life. We can choose to change the texture at any point. Take a deep breath, stop for a cup of tea, smile at someone, think of something that brings you joy, plan a dream. *"Be here now"* is how Baba Ram Dass put it. This minute, experience the part of the journey you are in now.

Make this minute what you want for a lifetime. Alter the texture of your day in any way you choose, but recognize that the texture and the minute are yours.

THE LOST THINGS LAW

The philosophical positions we take in life, the way we see things, have a lot to do with our happiness and the happiness of those around us. I call these positions the laws of the universe. For example, the Lost Things Law.

There are people who believe you can go through a lifetime without losing anything, as long as you're careful and thoughtful. They actually believe that a child can get through elementary school without losing a jacket. But that's impossible unless the child is repressed. A truly creative child will lose two jackets. Now, you can make a child wear an old jacket to school. You can ask the child to contribute to replacing the jacket. It's important to teach responsibility. But don't assume that if the child were just more thoughtful, he or she wouldn't lose anything.

Understand and recognize the laws of the universe and don't get mad. The creative person who lives his or her life up to its full potential will lose thousands of things. We don't have control over lost things, only over how we perceive a loss and how we handle it.

GRACE

Changing the way we perceive incidents can also change the way we respond to them.

A few years ago, I decided to add a "ten percent grace factor" to my life, and it has resulted in tremendous changes, all positive.

Assume a ten percent grace factor in your life:

Assume you'll pay ten percent more than your share of a dinner check shared with friends. Grace in your friendships is certainly worth that.

Assume that the bargain you got will cost ten percent less somewhere else tomorrow. Grace reduces stress.

Assume that you'll get cheated about ten percent of the time and that you'll lose about ten percent of your property one way or another. It costs to add grace to your life. It's worth it.

When you travel in another culture, assume a twenty percent grace factor. Then if you feel cheated by a taxi driver or someone else, it won't ruin more than a few minutes of your trip. Traveling in other countries requires grace.

Public grace will, in private, reduce tension, improve your perception of the world, improve your relationships, and increase your joy.

You'll end up with more of everything.

NOISE

One of the major changes in our environment in the last several years is the amount of noise. There's been a tremendous increase, and that noise causes significant amounts of stress.

Now, you may not notice it; you may think your body has adjusted to this kind of noise level. Only when something alarming happens, an airplane going overhead, a truck going by, a chain saw on a Saturday morning, only then are you aware. But this noise is around all the time and it adds stress.

You don't notice it until you go deep into the forest, and then all of a sudden you can hear silence. Your body no longer has to defend itself against the stress of noise.

Recognize that noise can make you tense and irritable. You're more likely to yell at someone shortly after the plane has gone by overhead. Once you recognize it, work to reduce noise in your home, in your workplace, wherever you have control.

Take a quiet break, even if it means using earplugs, at least once a day so that you can feel that peace. See if you can reduce the amount of noise that you contribute to the environment. We all need moments of silence.

DEPRESSION

Depression can mean thoughts of suicide or it can mean just feeling down. All of us experience depression. How well you handle it determines your personal ratio of good and bad times. There will always be some bad days, there always will be losses, but you can reduce the number.

Depression is a signal that your life is out of balance. You have decided that you are not valuable enough to enjoy life. Find out how you are out of balance, and why.

Depression may immobilize you so that you feel like giving up. You can overcome this feeling by understanding that depression is a message to take time to grow and heal. Your pain is a demand that you take time for change.

There are many ways to say that out of pain comes growth and joy, but none of them bring real comfort when you are depressed. Accept the down time, learn from it, and it will pass and return less often. When depression lingers, or the pain becomes overwhelming, take action. Find a counselor to help you reassess your balance and rebuild your worth.

The pain you feel at one moment in time will not be there forever.

HELP

We all need help sometimes. When you are hurt or confused, first, talk to yourself. Check what your feelings are. We are rarely upset for the reason we think.

Then try talking to the other person involved, if someone is, or talk to a friend. You'll get a different perspective.

You can check out a relevant book from the library or buy a book from a bookstore. You may not find a solution, but you'll find some new ideas.

Think about joining a class. You can call your local community college or your community information line. There are classes on most of the things that we worry about.

If you still feel that you don't have a solution, consider joining a group that works on that particular problem. There is a support group for almost everything.

If you feel that your problem is staying with you, find a counselor. You can go for a single session or you can make a longer commitment. The important thing is that you do something. Don't just learn to live with the problem. There's a better alternative.

LETTING GO

We must learn to let go as easily as we grasp or we will find our hands full and our minds empty.

—LEO BUSCAGLIA
The Way of the Bull

The search for security is often marked by the collecting of things. They seem a fortress against need. We get caught up in the belief that "more is better."

Piles of objects often take more time to clean and store than they save. We exhaust ourselves taking care of our property and social roles.

How many things do you have stored away for the future, like squirrels with their nuts? If you were asked to give away one half, what would you keep? When you dream about a fire, what do you rescue in the house? Make a list. Figure out what is weight and what helps you float.

Do you know what you want, or just what you've been told to want?

Focus on creating and enjoying instead of acquiring and holding on.

Build up all your assets, including your health, capacity to love, and appreciation of life.

When you let go of the constant urge to acquire, what you truly need begins to flow into your life.

EXPECTATIONS

One of the teachings of Eastern religions is that our biggest problem is desire. Sadness comes from the disappointments of unmet desires.

Eastern philosophers say the problem is having the desires in the first place. They suggest we put our energy into eliminating expectations rather than satisfying them.

Somewhere within each of us is a balance point between expectation and satisfaction.

What are your expectations? Trace where they came from. Ask yourself why you have them and what is in them for you. Are these desires built on your needs or someone else's?

People rarely question their expectations. Instead, they question their personal adequacy. Evaluate what truly brings you satisfaction and peace and let the rest go.

WHAT DO YOU WANT?

Most of us don't know what we want. We live our whole lives doing what we think we should want or what we think other people want us to do, and then when we realize we haven't lived our dreams, we have regrets.

My father was like that. He worked very hard his whole life and then when he realized he'd done it for other people and hadn't lived his dreams, he thought it was too late.

Find out what you want now. Every day ask yourself the question, *"What do I want?"* Put down the things that come to mind. Do it quickly. Don't let the filters drop into place.

Write down whatever it is. A greenhouse, a better relationship with your mother, financial security, world peace. Do it every day for a week, then take that list and cross off everything on that list that isn't what you want.

Cross off what your mother wants, what your father wants, what your other relatives want, what your spouse wants, what your neighbor wants, what the other people in your profession want, so that the only thing you have left is what you want. Once you know what it is, then you can make plans to get it.

Make a treasure map with you at the beginning and what you want at the end.

Check your desires often. What we want changes. You need to know.

PEAK

How does it feel when you're at your peak? On a roll?
Centered? Strutting your stuff? It feels good! Take a minute
to remember the last time you felt that way. Recapture it
and describe it. Do any of these adjectives fit?

calm	vital
focused	effortless
committed	spontaneous
confident	satisfied
energized	transcendent

When you're not at your peak the alternatives are
usually panic or the blahs. Always know where you are and
then decide if you want to stay there. We all panic or tune
out at times. The point is that you get to make the choice. If
you opt for peak you can get there. Remember how it feels.
Then try to shift gears. You may have your own tech-
niques; these are the ones I use:

notice where I am	take a dream break
decide to change it	commit an optimistic act
take a break	clean something
go for my strength	sort something
call someone	write a thank you
touch someone	plant something
exercise	change my environment
find some humor	

Check how you feel and what you want. As Woody
Allen pointed out, *"Eighty percent of success in life is showing
up."*

LEARNING HOW TO LIVE

If you can spend a perfectly useless afternoon in a perfectly useless manner, you have learned how to live.

—LIN YUTANG
The Importance of Living

How is that for a challenge? Can you let go? Are you proud of your ability to do three things at once and never waste a minute? How many of us travel through life at top speed, never realizing we've missed it?

TIME

There is more to life than increasing its speed.

There was a time when I felt I had to rush to accomplish anything. Nothing could stop me. Not stop lights, traffic, mistakes. I was irritated at things that got in my way—lack of parking spaces, other drivers, missed buses—but nothing slowed me down.

I measured the quality of my life by the speed at which it passed and the number of things I could do.

Then I stopped. I began to question. How did I want to spend my time? What choices was I making? Who was running my life?

I decided I wanted to improve the quality of every moment of my life, especially the time I spent with people. People I met every day in my community. I wanted to be able to see and hear the beauty around me.

I started choosing peace over conflict. I asked myself what was truly important. I started to give myself time to enjoy, to feel. I started to give myself rewards for accomplishments instead of expectations of more to be done. My life changed. I now know who is making the choices, who is deciding on the rewards and punishments. I am the only one controlling my life and my perception of that life.

It's important to give yourself rewards for quality. When you finish something that's important to you, stop and appreciate yourself. One of the rewards I like is solitude; also flowers, time for music, a hot bath, a new book. Another is a chocolate eclair.

MIDDLES

I'm good at beginnings: optimistic, filled with energy, and full of possibilities. I'm not bad at endings: dignified, conciliatory, trying to go out with class—or at least silence. It's middles that are the problem.

In the middle of something time slows down, questions of meaning arise, lethargy competes with apathy. I ask, *"Why am I doing this?"* It's hard to stay in the middle.

You can start over, or end it. But the message in the middle is really one of balance. Confusion, ambivalence, conflict, and tension are doors that are constantly flying open. You're not sure which way to go, if not to another ending or beginning.

Most of life is in the middle.

MIDLIFE

We usually think about the problem of midlife crisis when it's happening to someone else. The temptation is to resist change—to hold onto the status quo. Don't. If you set up a barrier to change, you may get left in the past. Instead, encourage questions. See if you can help your partner find answers.

Agree to talk things over or find a counselor. Be independent. Don't try to hold on. Try to stretch and grow. Invest in changes that both of you can share. The fear of change is the fear that we can't also grow. Push for your own growth, and you won't feel anxious about the future.

Midlife crisis, whether it seems positive or negative, comes from the heart. It's the desire to have a full life. Push for growth in yourself, and the resolution will be positive. It may not be what you planned years ago, but it will be positive nonetheless.

DANCE OF LIFE

One of the frustrations we all face is thinking that we can get everything done. You make a list and assume you can get to the bottom of it. But, by then, there's another list. There always will be. That's the process of life.

The same thing happens when we grow and change. I call it the "Dance of Life"—two steps forward and one step back. We think we've solved something and it turns up again. We "dance" as individuals and as a society.

There will always be change, there will always be new challenges. We'll be handling them, but the Dance of Life will be the same. It's the body's way of stabilizing and reducing stress. It's how our society keeps its balance. Time to stabilize before the next leap forward.

Expect the dance, celebrate the forward steps, be ready for the step back. Recognize and move with the rhythm in your life and in your culture.

SUNSHINE

I used to find it hard to fully enjoy a beautiful summer day. I was tense if I had to work inside; I worried that the sun would go away before I had had enough. Then the gray season would come and I wouldn't have enough sun to last.

Then I started bottling sunshine. Go outside, soak up the sun and fill quart jars in your mind. When the shelves are full, you'll be secure. Next winter, when the weather gets you down, just open a jar, pour it over yourself, and relax.

MISTAKES

How many mistakes did you make this week? A full life requires thousands of mistakes if you plan to live up to your creative potential.

When we are children, adults try to talk us out of making mistakes and we get confused. They are referring to life-threatening mistakes, but we think they mean everything.

Check how open you are to mistakes. Can you stand it? Can you laugh? Do you shy away from things you might not do well? Do you laugh at people who seem clumsy or naive? Do you grit your teeth when someone you love makes a mistake? Are you under the illusion that everyone is watching you and keeping score?

Start counting your mistakes on a daily basis and try to increase them by ten percent. That will require you to stretch and grow. Try not mentioning other people's mistakes. Take risks; be tolerant of yourself and others.

Congratulate others on the risks they take; admire their courage. You'll have more pleasure and be much closer to what you want to be. Mistakes are the dues of a good and full life. Stretch and enjoy.

TRANSITIONS

Give yourself transition time at the end of the formal work day. It's too hard to shift abruptly from one sphere to the next. You leave part of yourself behind.

There are lots of ways to make the transition, to take off the masks you might have put on when you went out the door in the morning.

Sit in your office and review the day before you head out for the traffic jam. Pull into a park or by the side of the road and watch the sky change light. Go for a walk before you enter your home or gently stroll through the shopping for dinner ritual.

You can also make the shift once you get home. Take care of the crises, if there are any, then find a quiet place to sit, or read the paper, or sweep the front sidewalk. Give yourself at least a few minutes. Make a contract with the person you live with for "transition time."

Take time to make peace with your day and renew your energy for your home and the people you love.

RISK

Studies of people who report high well-being in their fifties and sixties indicate that they have lived lives that involved personal risks. They are not people whose lives have been calm and predictable. A life under tight control sometimes produces quiet desperation.

High well-being is a life that has depth and quality. Risks, losses, problems, and tragedy add pain to a life. That pain becomes a teacher. We learn; the pain gives us no choice.

Richard Bach, in his book *Illusions,* stated, *"Every tragedy has a gift for you in its hands,"* but it is hard sometimes to see that gift. When you are too busy to acknowledge your pain, when you deny it, you still feel the pain but you lose the gift.

Resistance expands pain. Instead, lean into it and move through it. Give yourself time to grieve, to grow, and to feel life.

Celebrate the life lived for all it offers. Allow for the deepening of your personal awareness and the clearing of your values.

OTHER PATHS

To talk in public, to think in solitude, to read and to hear, to inquire and answer inquiries, is the business of a scholar.

—SAMUEL JOHNSON
Letters to the Earl of Chesterfield

I always wanted to be a scholar, somehow searching for truth. I didn't know what I would do with it if I found any, but the search was bound to be exciting. I felt a passion for "knowledge" and a physical thrill whenever I walked onto a university campus. I was captivated by the search and the part I might play in it.

I stayed many years, and wrote many articles before I realized that something was wrong. I had missed a path somewhere. I felt isolated from "my truths," I felt cut off from reality, from the community I was part of. I felt myself growing smaller and tighter. I felt trapped in a shell that, while viewed by some as an elite shell, was nevertheless a powerful filter obscuring my vision.

I decided to leave the university. I saw another path, and it has made all the difference.

Allow yourself to see other paths; there will be many. Allow yourself the freedom to choose more than one life-work. Allow yourself to move when your heart moves.

WINDOWS

When the present seems hopelessly bogged down, I turn, for a few moments, to the future.

I feel an intuitive attraction pulling me. I can see and feel the future. I know where we will travel if we move beyond our current life-patterns.

Crises always preceded perceptual transformation. It's as if we need to be bumped into an ability to see clearly.

The choices seem obvious, but you must make the commitment.

connection, not elitism
empowerment, not power over others
community, not isolation
participation, not observation
self-discipline, not letting go
touching, not sex
intuition as well as logic
humor, not hopelessness
grace, not control
optimism, not pessimism
meaning as well as comfort
spirit, not emptiness

Open the window of the future that is within you. Peek out, stretch, lean toward it, and prepare to tumble through.

If you want happiness
  for an hour—take a nap.
If you want happiness
  for a day—go fishing.
If you want happiness
  for a month—get married.
If you want happiness
  for a year—inherit a fortune.
If you want happiness
  for a lifetime—help someone else.

—CHINESE PROVERB

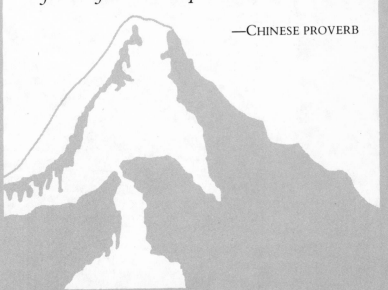

CONNECTIONS

A human being is a part of the whole, called by us "Universe," a part limited in time and space. He experiences himself, his thoughts and feelings as something separated from the rest—a kind of optical illusion of his consciousness. This delusion is a kind of prison for us, restricting us to our personal desires and to affection for a few persons nearest to us. Our task must be to free ourselves from this prison by widening our circle of compassion to embrace all living creatures and the whole of nature in its beauty. Nobody is able to achieve this completely, but the striving for such achievement is in itself a part of the liberation and foundation for inner security.

—ALBERT EINSTEIN
Albert Einstein, The Human Side

POP

The word *pop*, as in pop art and pop music, used to bother me. *Pop* meant *popular*, and I went along with the view that things were valuable only if they were rare or hard to understand.

The word *public* had a similar ring. It meant people who achieved less. I learned at the universities that *public* meant *mediocre*, the "public press" or "the masses."

I questioned this elitism because I sensed its inherent cruelty, but I didn't see then that it limits knowledge and awareness. Elitism is a dense filter.

I began to realize that *pop* means *public*, "of the people"—something lots of people can enjoy and understand. It means language that is clear instead of "jargon" that maintains separation. It means ideas that are shared, not information guarded as professional secrets.

Now, I find myself called a pop psychologist. (Actually, I am a pop anthropologist.) I know why I made the choice. I am of the public, part of the community. I don't want to be separate anymore. I've fallen in love with the open door, the chance to learn, the spirit among us all.

I laugh at the thought and tingle at the possibility that I am becoming a pop person.

CHAUTAUQUA

I'm thinking of making a change. It's time for the return of chautauquas. *Chautauqua* is a Seneca Indian word that means, in part, a gathering of the clan.

Chautauquas were old-time tent shows that moved across America—a series of talks to open up people's minds, to share thoughts and information.

The chautauquas were pushed aside by the faster pace of radio and television. Our national consciousness moves faster now, but it seems less deep.

I would like to slow down, to dig deeper into old values, into those thoughts that have become burdened and stale with platitudes.

Can you listen to a slower dialogue? Can you exchange the quick surface sketch for a deeper look? Can you ask, as you watch television and listen to the radio, *"What is good?"*, not, *"What is new?"*

We sometimes feel we have too much to do to slow down and listen, to take a closer look at the quality of the journey. We forget to ask, *"What is important?"*

There is still time to slip into the tent and talk.

Inspired by Zen and the Art of Motorcycle Maintenance, *by Robert Pirsig*

RESULTS

Choose to have fun. Fun creates enjoyment. Enjoyment invites participation. Participation focuses attention. Attention expands awareness. Awareness promotes insight. Insight generates knowledge. Knowledge facilitates action. Action yields results.

—OSWALD B. SHALLOW

ABUNDANCE

That which we bless multiplies. This is an inescapable spiritual law of the universe. The one who chooses the spiritual pathway to success and happiness must be willing to shift from an attitude of lack to one of thanksgiving in order to take the first step.

—Reverend Jim Munson

We have so much, yet many Americans feel dissatisfied. Somehow the full table, symbol of abundance to the pilgrims, is not enough. We yearn for something far beyond material satisfaction.

Find your place in history this Thanksgiving by stretching beyond your table. Celebrate your survival by offering peace and sharing with your neighbors.

Make the shift from an illogical feeling of lack to the recognition of abundance. Invite the Spirit to your feast, and prepare to feed the world.

PUBLIC GRACE

When I was in Japan I was struck by a phenomenon that I'll call public grace. Wherever I went, even on busy sidewalks, I was treated with grace and respect. The gesture of greeting that the Japanese use is not a bow of deference, it's a bow of respect. *"I don't know you, but I respect you."*

It reminded me of a similar gesture in India which translates, *"I respect the God within you."*

Wherever I went, whether I was making a purchase in a store, receiving service in hotels or restaurants, or walking on the sidewalks or in parks, people were courteous and helpful.

I felt very welcome and very safe, even though I didn't speak the language. I felt safer than in any other country in the world.

In the northwest United States we have a lot more space for people than they have in Japan, but I'd like to vote for a little more public grace between strangers, when you're receiving service, or among friends.

It's up to you to set a model and give other people the chance to discover the grace within them and between us.

OPTIMISTIC ACTS

What choices are you making in your perception of the events around you? We choose how we view our times. There is a pinch of pessimism in our culture now. Counter it with small acts of optimism.

Pick up a piece of litter that isn't yours. Show some extra grace on the freeway. Give to your food bank. Smile at a child who is in your way. Help someone you know. Help someone you don't know.

The accumulation of small, optimistic acts produces quality in our culture and in your life. Our culture resonates in tense times to individual acts of grace. What's your choice?

COMMUNITY

Above all, a city needs a soul if it is to become a true home for human beings. You, the people, must give it this soul.

—POPE JOHN PAUL II

You are, whether with reluctance or with commitment, a unit of this community.

The community you live in is not an entity separate from your life. It is a representation of your life. You are the individual unit, the multiple of which is us.

Sometimes we feel alienated from our culture, as if it moved separately from the people who compose it. It cannot move without us. We shape its values and its quality at each and every moment.

How are your values shaping your community? Stop a moment and imagine all the people whom you identify as part of your community. Decide what your contribution to their quality of life will be. The quality of your life will be closely attuned to the quality of theirs.

VOTING

All the candidates and their supporters have been reminding us to vote. They talk about responsibility. They talk about caring, about our community. You may say you don't care. You may feel guilty. But don't vote out of guilt.

Vote out of optimism. It's an optimistic act to be involved in your community. I think it's essential to your well-being and to your peace of mind. If you drive to work, you may see people holding campaign signs. Even though they probably got up at 6 A.M., they're cheerful and excited, especially the children. They sense that they're involved in something important.

Get out your newspaper, get your sample ballot, choose your candidate, choose your issues, get help if you need it. Call your candidate's office if you want a ride to the polls, or get an absentee ballot ahead of time.

Vote out of optimism, not pessimism. Choose community over isolation. Whatever the outcome, you'll be giving something good to yourself, and maybe to the rest of us as well.

THE SPIRIT

God is too big to fit inside one religion.

—SONDRA BARNES
Life Is the Way It Is

The future requires openness to all spiritual knowledge. You may prefer one religion, but there are many paths to the center and we need all the help we can get.

People who believe there is only one path limit themselves. They find safety in spiritual rigidity. They memorize phrases and mindlessly repeat them, confusing faith with obedience. They threaten damnation, they hurl insults in the name of God. They cannot feel the love of the prophets they quote. They preach limits in the realm of the unlimited.

The message of the spirit throughout the world is the same. It is a message of love, tolerance, compassion, respect, optimism, and a profound understanding of the meaning of community.

RENAISSANCE

Renaissance is a wonderful, rich word that means revival, a new birth. It is the spirit of new life and new values. Here are some ways to bring yourself a touch of the spirit:

Express love to a family member or a stranger in a way that does not involve money.

Give the present of your time and attention to a child.

Take time to reach toward your own spiritual center in whatever way touches you. Give yourself love.

Make one contribution to peace within your family, among your friends, and in your world.

Choose peace of mind over conflict.

MULTIPLES

There is more ambivalence in our lives now than there was in the past. There is more confusion and there are more questions of meaning.

In part this is because we live in a multiple-option world. Once we pass basic survival, the options for Americans seem endless—whether it's choosing a flavor of ice cream, whom to live with, or what to believe in.

For those of us raised on Neopolitan ice cream and marriage, it's intimidating. Don't try to buy a stereo or a car without a sixteen-year-old along to provide advice. There are too many alternatives and variations.

The negative is that life is more complex and decisions wear us out. The positive is that the choices are now ours. We are more tolerant of others who choose differently. We accept a wider spectrum of love, faith, and style.

There is more individual responsibility for what we are and the way we touch our communities.

Next time you feel overwhelmed, breathe in deeply the freedom, accept the responsibility, and remember the joy that can go with it. You have the ability to make a unique, individual choice. If it is good, it is yours; and if not, you can choose differently next time.

LAWS OF THE UNIVERSE

Let's talk about the laws of the universe again. It's important to understand how the world works. Sometimes we make false assumptions, and then get frustrated.

Let's discuss the law pertaining to toilet paper rolls. There are some of you out there who think that anyone in a household can be taught to put the toilet paper on the toilet paper roll. That's not true. The law actually says that in any given household only one person will voluntarily do this task.

I found out that I was the designated person in my house, and I tried to fight it. I even hired a housekeeper two afternoons a week, and I taught her how to put the toilet paper on the roll, and she nodded.

I left her notes, but in two years she has never once put the toilet paper on the toilet paper roll. I have finally accepted the law of the universe, that I'm the designated person, and it has brought me peace of mind.

STRENGTH

We have too many men of science, too few men of God. We have grasped the mystery of the atom and rejected the Sermon on the Mount . . . Ours is a world of nuclear giants and ethical infants. We know more about war than we know about peace, more about killing than we know about living.

—GENERAL OMAR N. BRADLEY
Address given on Armistice Day, 1948

There is a fear of peace that I do not understand. Witness the old epithet "peaceniks," the association of peace with weakness. We mistake kindness for weakness in individuals, too.

Gandhi found the essence of Christianity to be gentleness, the exaltation of means over ends.

Using violence, against us or them, to achieve peace is like beating children to get them to be good. It only works in the short term.

Believe in peace, think peace, live peace. Be a building-block of peace. Make it the center of your strength.

HEART AND MIND

If the world kept a journal, many of the entries would be conversations concerning the advancement of scientific knowledge and its importance to humanity.

I offer the following conversation as an added entry.

"And what is as important as knowledge?" asked the mind.

"Caring," answered the heart.

—FLAVIA WEEDN

THE FUTURE

Unit Alert! The future will be what you are. It is not a separate thing, any more than a community is.

Marilyn Ferguson in her book *The Aquarian Conspiracy* writes about our need to recognize that we "breathe together"—the root meaning of the word *conspiracy*. *Aquarian* refers to the "new age," the age of "enlightenment." We are forever seeking "The Age of Aquarius."

I once defined *enlightenment* as being able to go to your own home and feel comfortable. Nirvana, ecstasy, paradise are not found on the tops of mountains in Tibet, although it's a beautiful trek. Enlightenment is found only within your own home.

Our past is not our potential. In any hour, with all the stubborn teachers and healers of history who called us to be our best selves, we can liberate the future. One by one, we can re-choose—to awaken. To leave the prison of our conditioning, to love, to turn homeward. To conspire with and for each other. Awakening brings its own assignments, unique to each of us, chosen by each of us. Whatever you may think about yourself, and however long you may have thought it, you are not just you. You are a seed, a silent promise. You are the conspiracy.

—MARILYN FERGUSON
The Aquarian Conspiracy

PEACE

Peace is a unit-by-unit phenomenon; it builds slowly. The feelings that bring peace and the behavior that is peace develop in small, individual steps.

It's important to work toward world peace, but the seed of its reality lies within each world citizen.

Peace within is a difficult concept for those who are distressed, hungry, or afraid. When you are well-fed and safe, it is a journey through levels of consciousness.

Until you achieve peace with yourself and your values, you cannot move to the next level of awareness.

Peace within our lives will extend beyond our lives.

The journey of a thousand miles
begins and ends with one step.

—LAO TSU
Tao Te Ching

Acknowledgments

P. vii: From "Little Gidding," in *Four Quartets* by T. S. Eliot. Copyright 1943 by T.S. Eliot; renewed 1971 by Esme Valerie Eliot. Reprinted by permission of Harcourt Brace Jovanovich, Inc.

P. 9: From *The Road Less Traveled,* copyright © 1976 by M. Scott Peck, M.D. Reprinted by permission of Simon & Schuster, Inc.

P. 16: Quote from Gerald May from personal communication with the author.

P. 18: Quote from Ken Wapnick from personal communication with the author.

P. 25: From "Judy Garland and the Global Death Wish, or, How to Stop Worrying and Enjoy Stolichnaya." Reprinted by permission of Tom Robbins.

P. 28: From *Reverence for Life* by Albert Schweitzer, copyright © 1969 by Rhena Eckert-Schweitzer. Reprinted by permission of Harper & Row Publishers, Inc.

P. 33: From *Leaves of Grass* by Walt Whitman. Edited and with an introduction by Malcolm Cowley. Copyright © 1959 by The Viking Press Incorporated. Reprinted by permission of Viking Penguin Incorporated.

P. 40: "The $700 Guru," reprinted by permission of Sharon Creedon (Rose of Sharon).

P. 49: "The Rose," by Amanda McBroom, © 1977, 1979 Warner-Tamerlane Publishing Corp., Hollywood Allstar Music, Third Story Music Inc. All rights reserved. Used by permission.

P. 79: Reprinted by permission of Rev. Ernest J. Forks and *The New Times*.

P. 91: Quote from David Burns from *Psychology Today,* November 1980.

P. 115: From Helen Dukas and Banesh Hoffman, *Albert Einstein, The Human Side: New Glimpses from his Archives.* Copyright © 1979 by the estate of Albert Einstein. Published by Princeton University Press.

P. 130: From *The Aquarian Conspiracy: Personal and Social Transformation in the 1980s.* Copyright © 1980 Marilyn Ferguson. Reprinted by permission of J. P. Tarcher, Inc.

About the Author

A Ph.D. in cultural anthropology who also holds master's degrees in history and psychology, Jennifer James was for twelve years a full-time faculty member of the psychiatry department of the University of Washington before she committed herself to a career in community service and communications. A weekly columnist for the *Seattle Times* for more than twelve years, she hosted a daily radio talkshow that ranked among the region's top-rated programs.

Dr. James is the author of *Visions from the Heart, Success Is the Quality of Your Journey, Windows, You Know I Wouldn't Say This If I Didn't Love You, How to Survive the Next 100 Years, Women and the Blues: Passions that Hurt, Passions that Heal,* and *Life Is a Game of Choice.* She lectures worldwide to school, university, and professional groups, including ITT, IBM, Boeing, and the Young Presidents' Organization. She lives in Seattle, Washington.

Share Jennifer James with a friend.

Jennifer James has helped thousands to change their attitudes from the conventional yardstick of success—and to lead happier, more peace-filled lives. Reward a friend with Dr. James's writings on how to stop the grind and share the moments of pleasure and warmth.

Visions: In this book of meditations James takes her readers on a step-by-step journey to self-discovery and personal change. Trade paperback. 144 pages.

Success Is the Quality of Your Journey: 120 insights and ideas on subjects such as risk, solitude, aging, and relationships. Trade paperback. 144 pages.

Windows: 120 more essays on the topics of day-to-day living, intimacy, heroic acts, traveling (including the author's journey to Nepal), and more. Trade paperback. 160 pages.

You Know I Wouldn't Say This If I Didn't Love You: How to Defend Yourself Against Verbal Zaps and Zingers: Filled with nitty-gritty advice for both the giver and getter of criticism, James's book will help readers defend themselves from—and laugh at—the absurd and harmful things we say to each other. Illustrated. Trade paperback. 144 pages.

Ask for these titles at your local bookstore, or order by mail today.

Use this coupon, or write to:
Newmarket Press, 18 East 48th Street, New York, NY 10017

Please send me:
_____copies of *Visions*, in paperback, @ $9.95 each;
_____copies of *Success*, in paperback, @ $9.95 each;
_____copies of *Windows*, in paperback, @ $9.95 each;
_____copies of *You Know I Wouldn't Say This*, in paperback,
     @ $10.95 each.

Please include applicable sales tax, and add $2.00 for postage and handling (plus $1.00 for each additional item ordered)—check or money order only. Please allow 4-6 weeks for delivery. Prices and availability are subject to change.

Enclosed is a check or money order, payable to Newmarket Press, in the amount of $_____.

Name_____

Address _____

City/State/Zip _____

Companies, professional groups, clubs, and other organizations may qualify for special terms on quantity purchases of these titles. For more information, please phone or write: Special Sales Department, Newmarket Press, 18 East 48th Street, New York, N.Y. 10017 (212) 832-3575.